NEPHROLOGY

for kids

Medical School
FOR KIDS™

Copyright © 2022 Betty Nguyen & Brandon Pham

All rights reserved. No part of this book may be reproduced or used in any manner without the prior written permission of the copyright owner, except for the use of brief quotations in a book review.

First paperback edition December 2022

Book design by Betty Nguyen & Brandon Pham

ISBN 978-1-957557-08-3 (paperback)

Printed in the United States of America

Published by Black Phoenix Press

www.mdforkids.org

Disclaimer: Contents of this book are for informational purposes only. No material in this book is intended to provide, or be a substitute for, professional medical advice.

To the friends and family who have supported and loved us unconditionally, and to the mentors who have guided and taught us more than we could have imagined:

Thank you.

Betty & Brandon

Medical School FOR KIDS™

Nephrology

(neh-FRAA-luh-jee)

the branch of medicine concerned with the study and treatment of disorders and diseases of the kidneys

Medical School FOR KIDS™

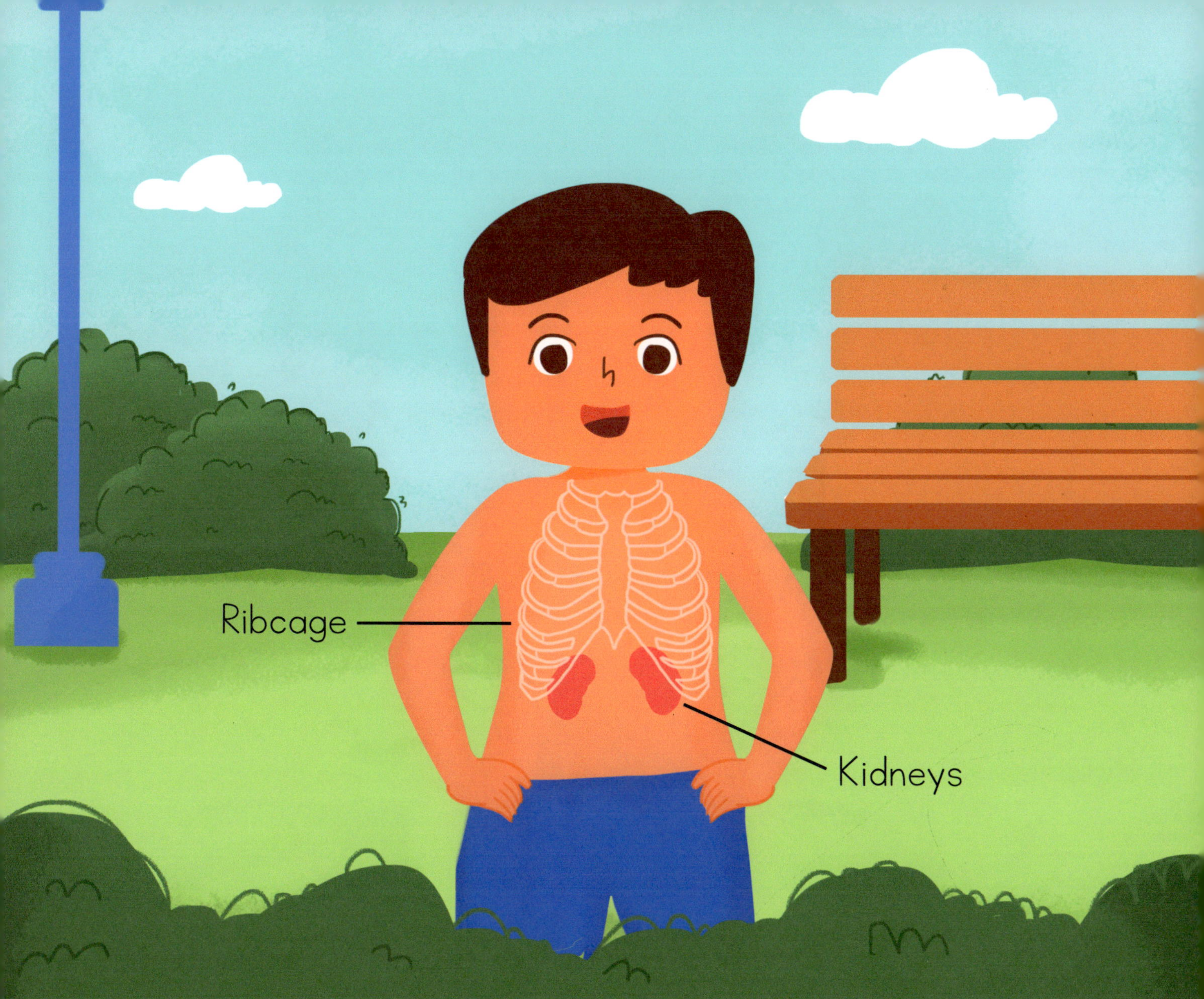

The **kidneys** are two bean-shaped organs located just below the ribcage.

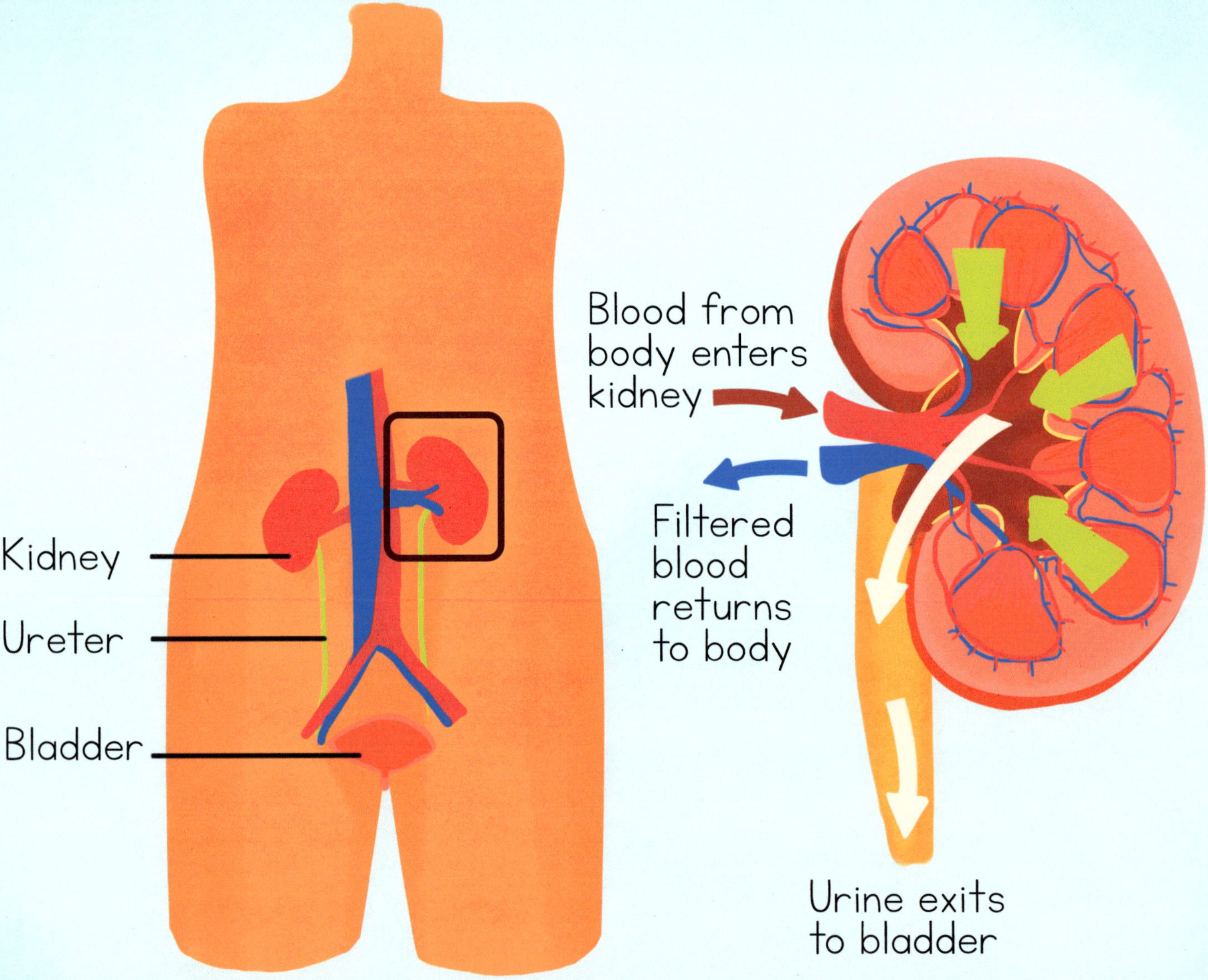

The kidneys filter blood, removing wastes and extra fluid from the body to make **urine** (pee)!

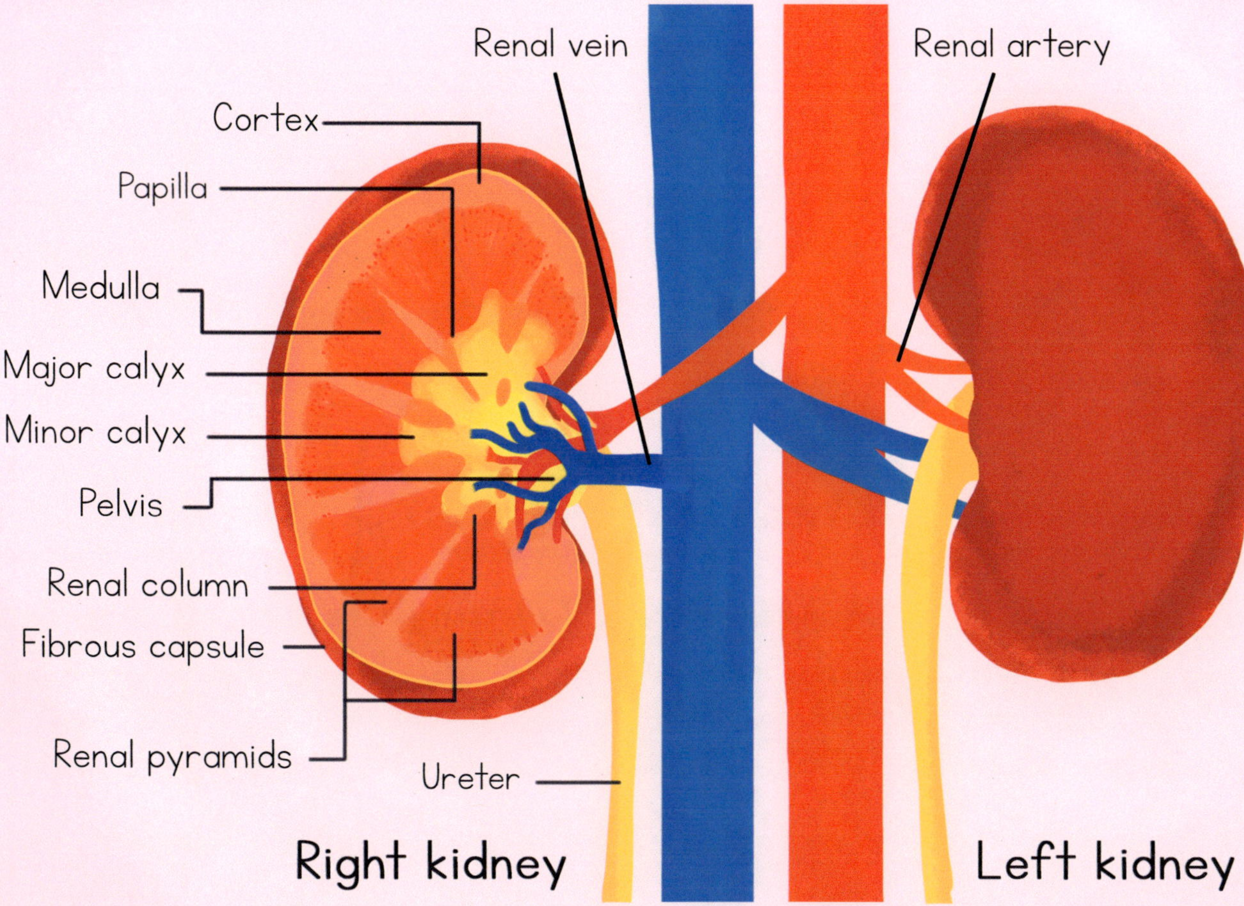

Blood that needs to be filtered first travels to the kidneys through the **renal arteries**.

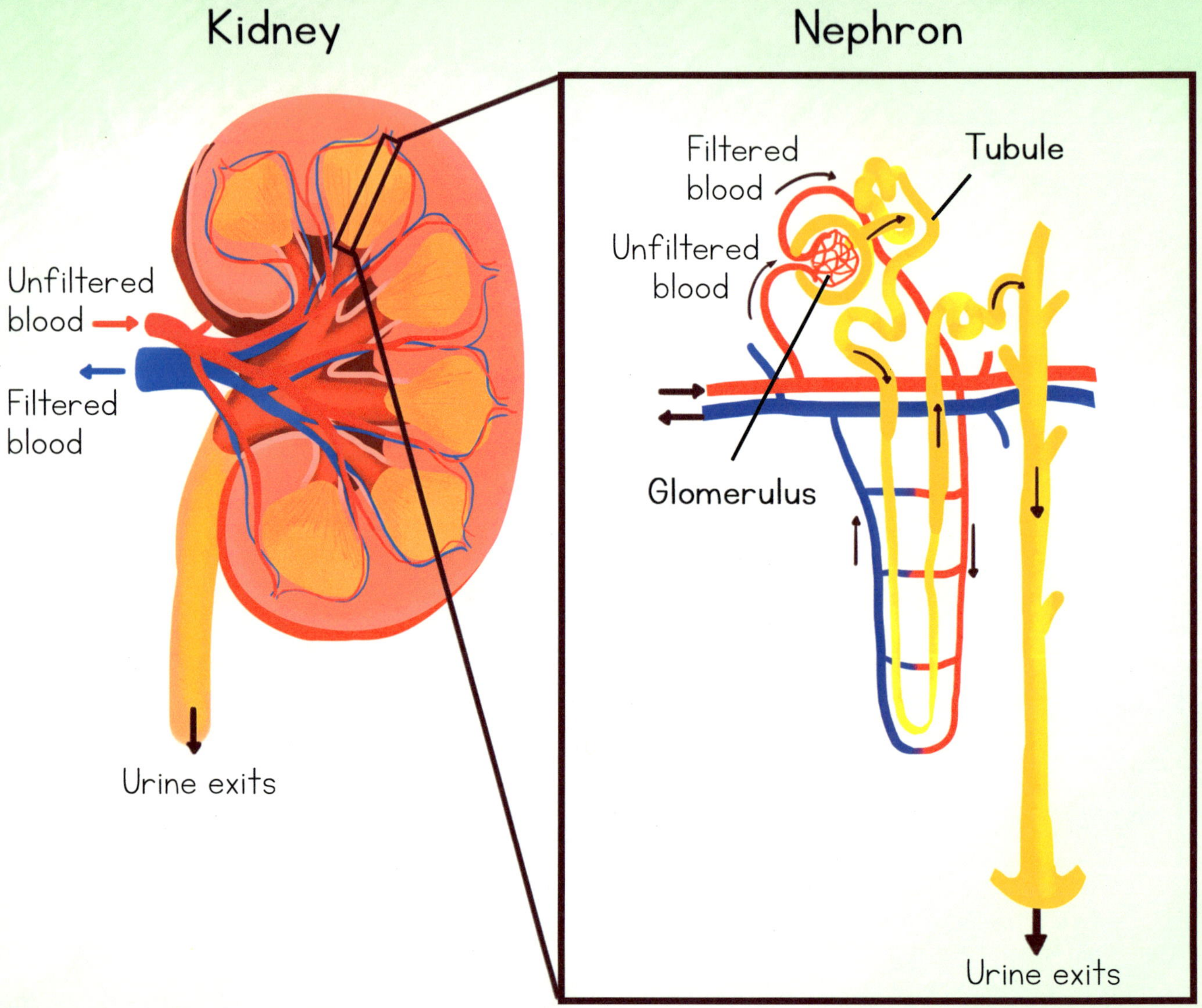

The kidneys are made of tiny cells called **nephrons**, which each has a **glomerulus** that filters urine and a **tubule** that collects urine.

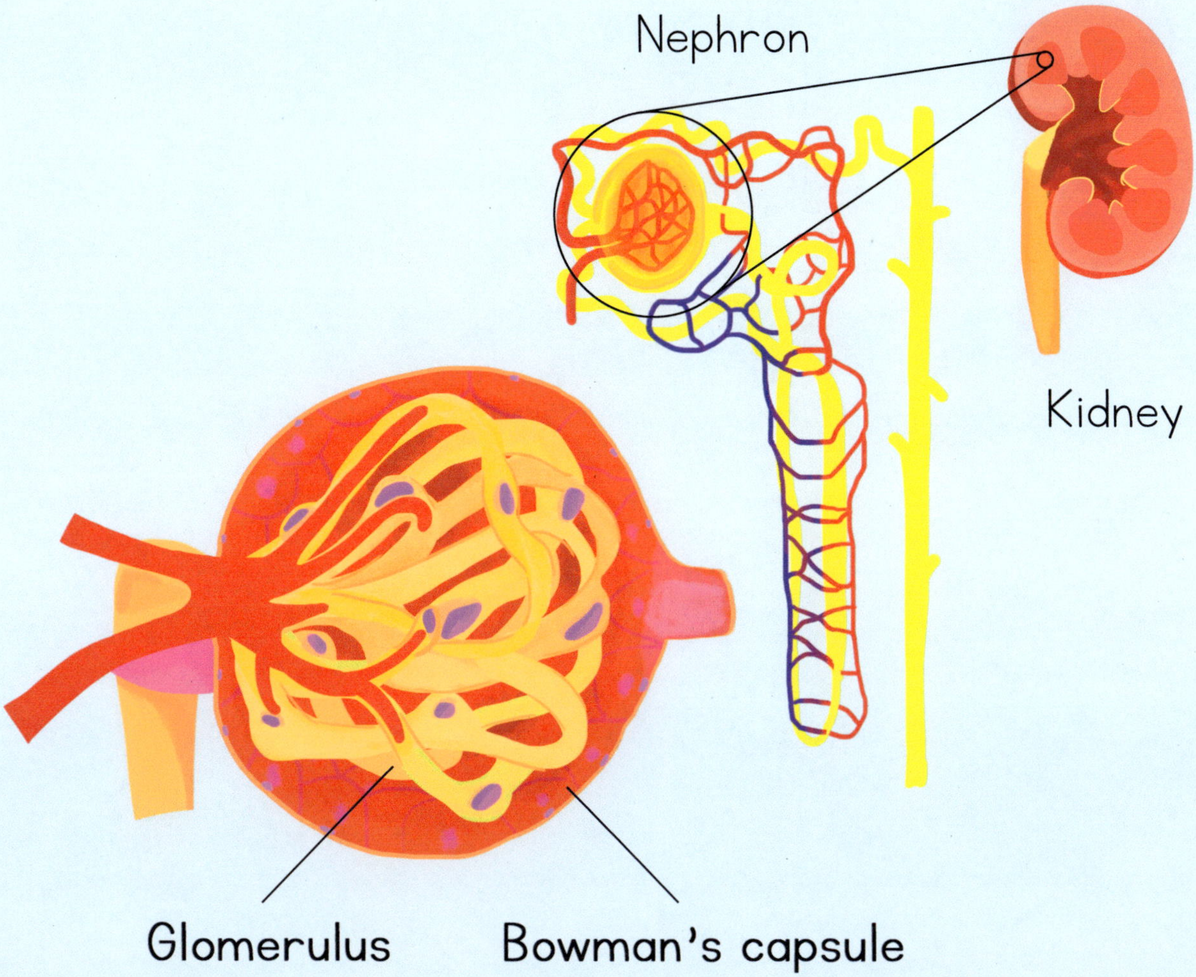

The **glomerulus** is a cluster of blood vessels where wastes are filtered out of the blood into the first part of the tubule, called **Bowman's capsule**.

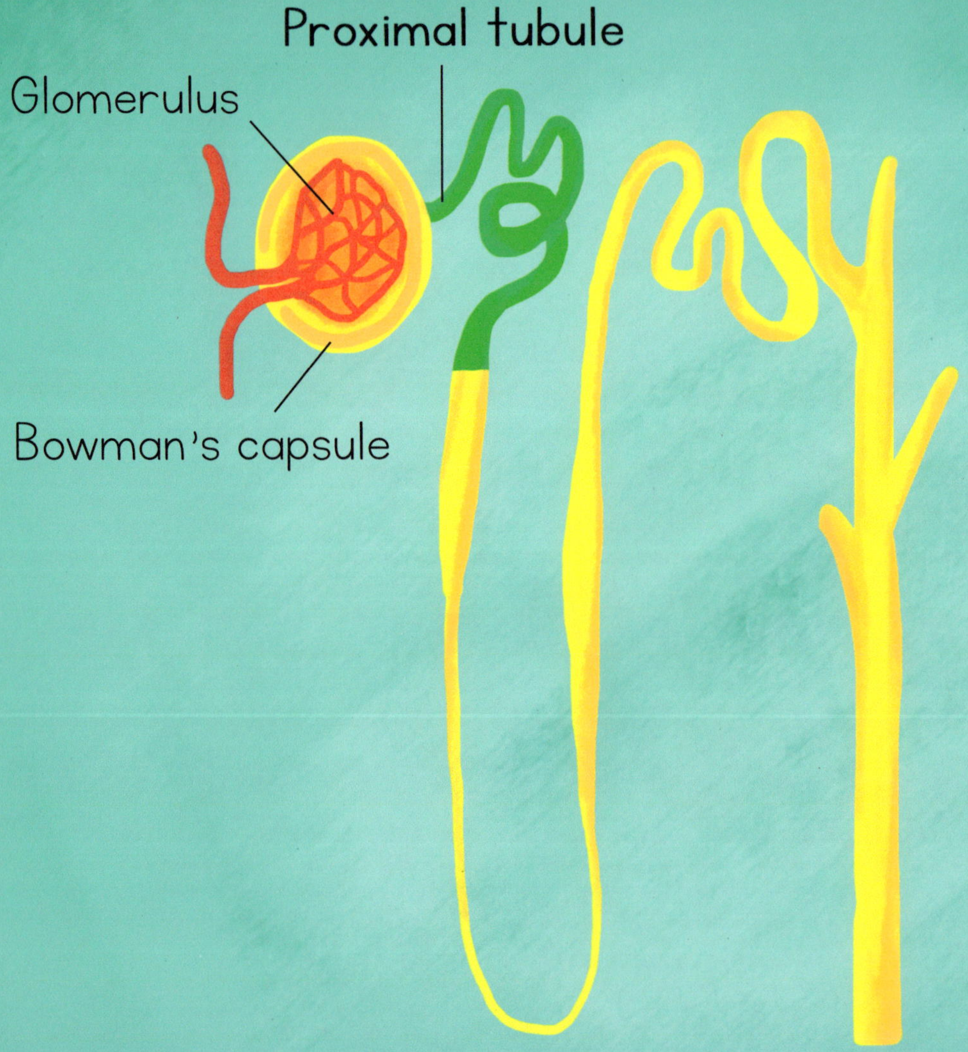

The next part of the tubule is the **proximal tubule**. Here, salts, sugar, and water are reabsorbed back into the blood.

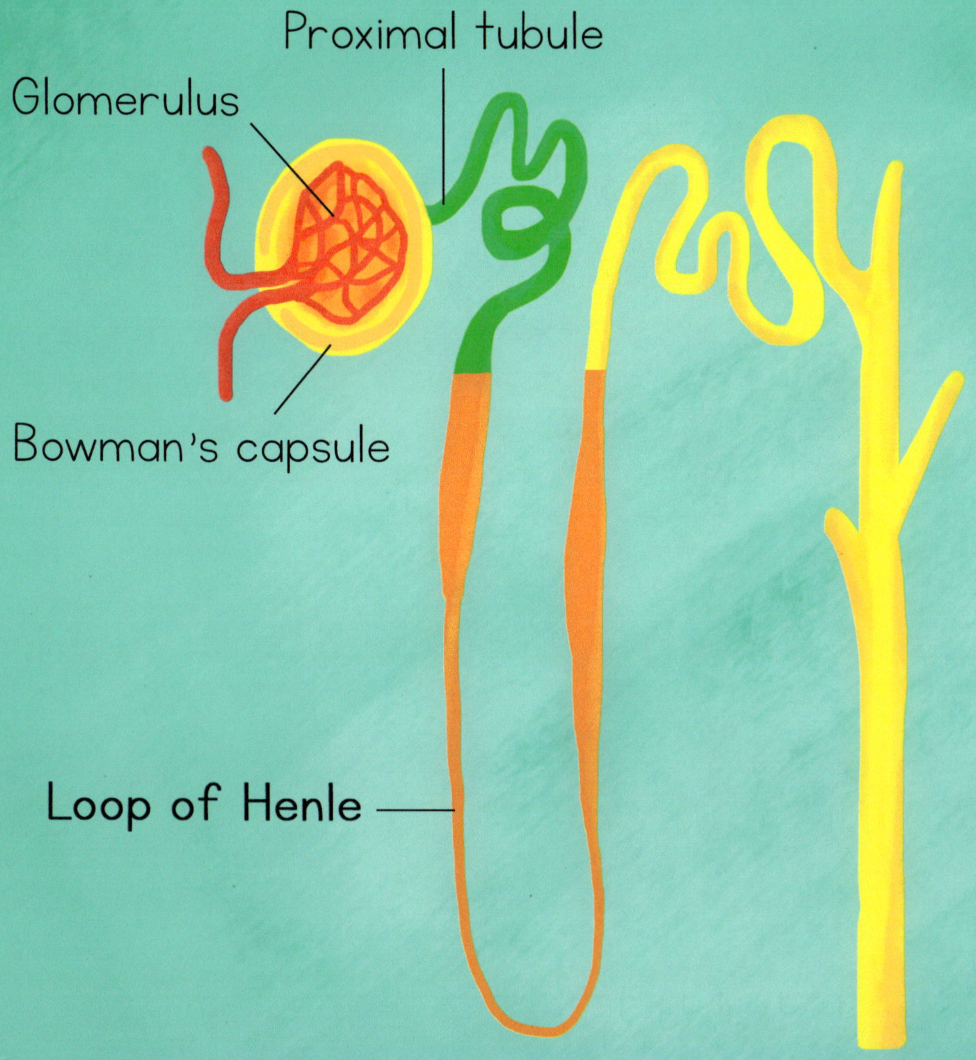

The next part of the tubule is the **loop of Henle**, where more water and salts are reabsorbed back into the blood.

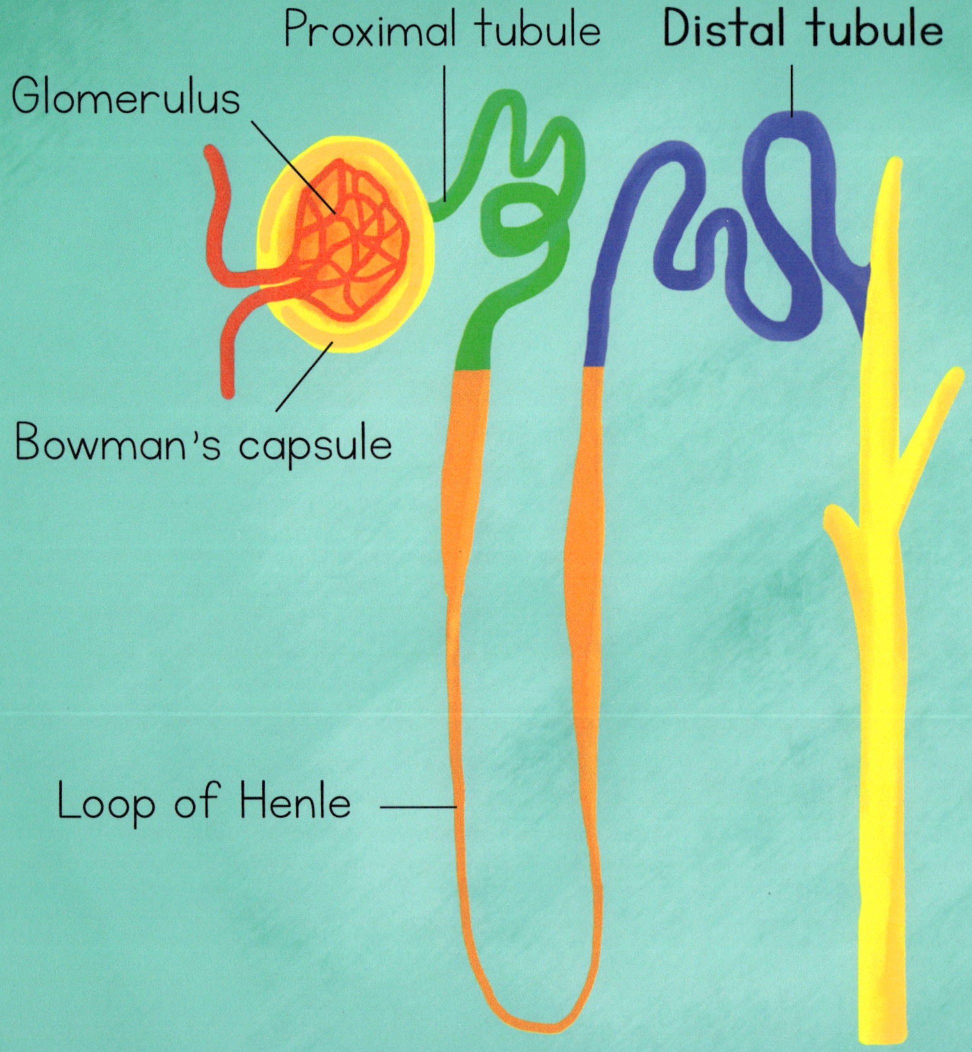

The next part of the tubule is the **distal tubule**, which helps fine-tune the amount of salts in our urine.

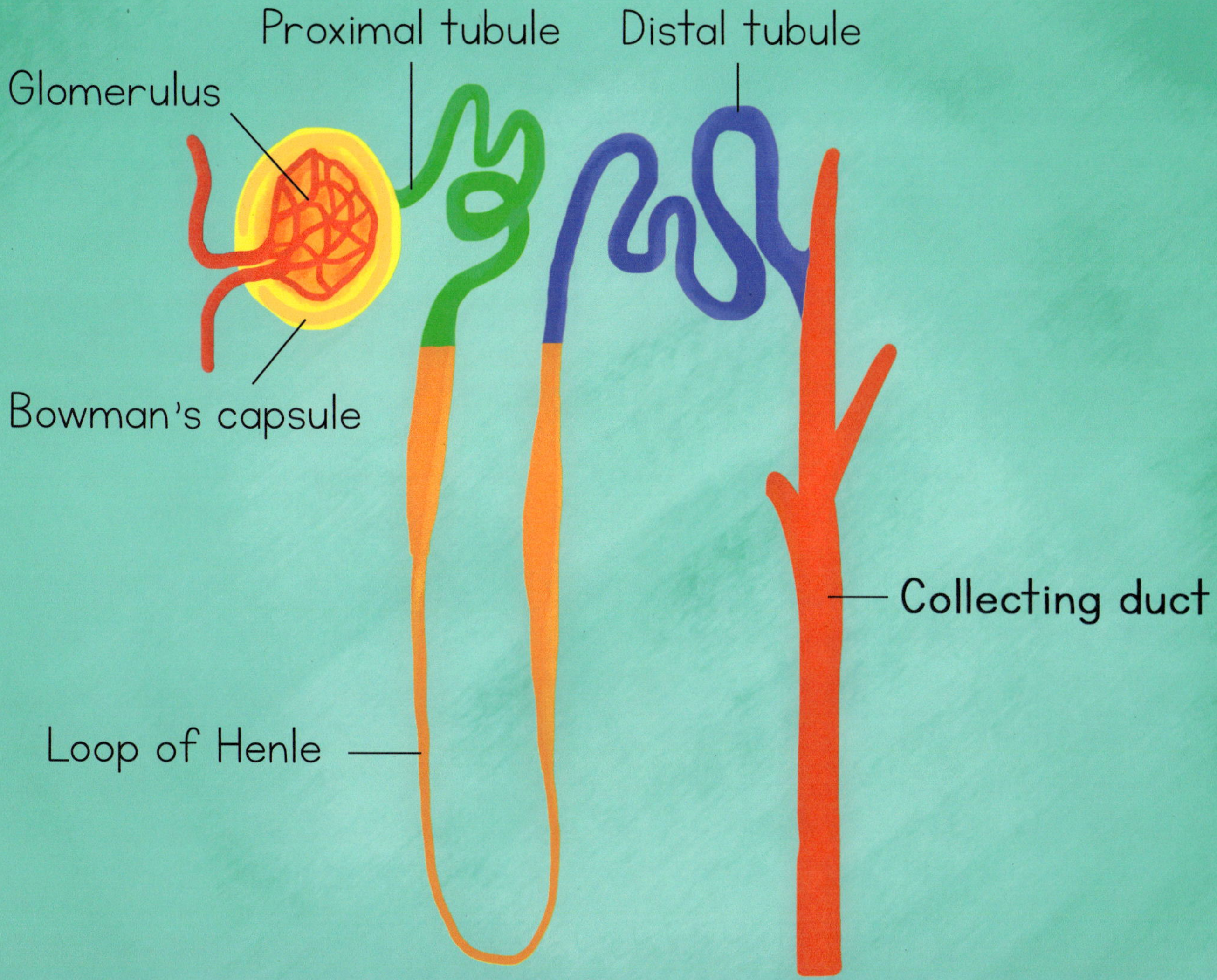

The last part of the tubule is the **collecting duct**, which helps fine-tune the amount of water in our urine.

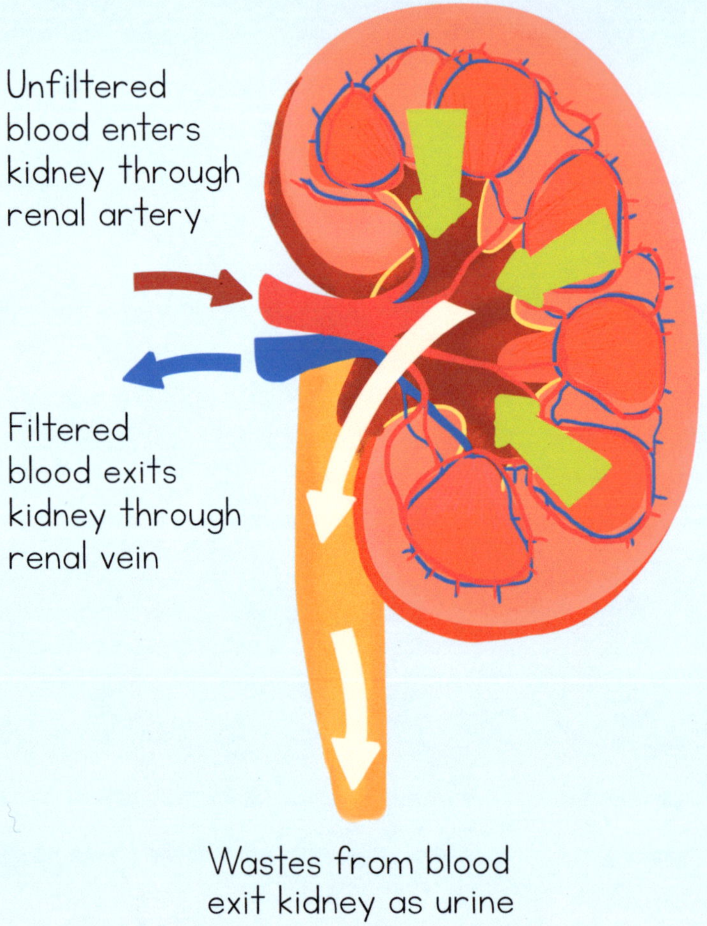

After wastes from the blood have been removed into the urine, filtered blood is ready to return to the body through the **renal vein**.

Urine color

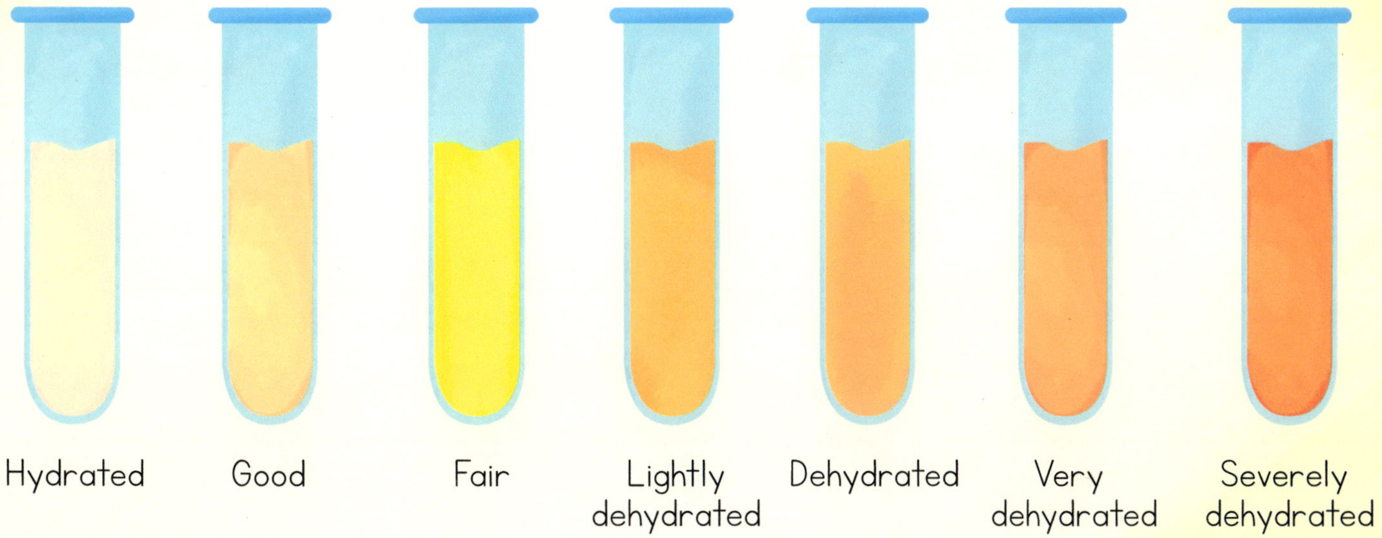

The amount of water we drink affects our urine color. When we drink enough water, our urine should have a light yellow color.

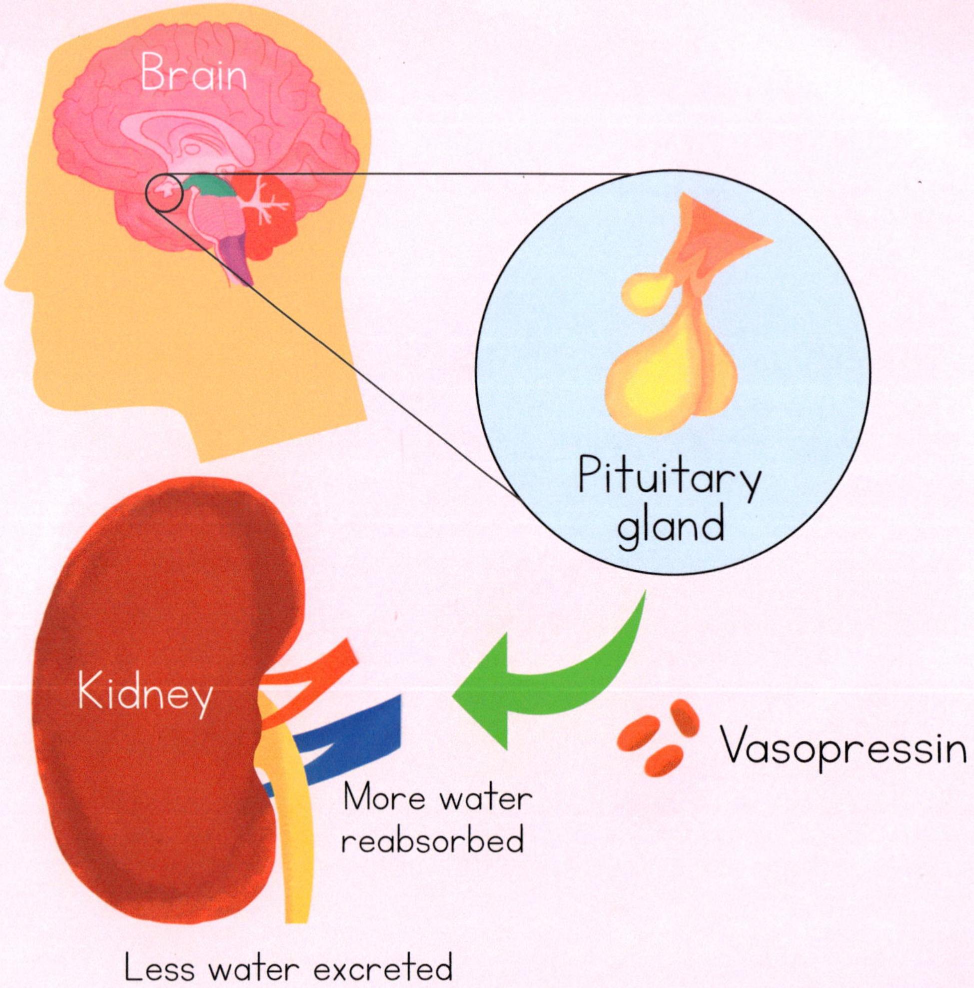

When we don't drink enough water, our urine gets darker because our brain releases a hormone (**vasopressin**) that tells our kidneys to reabsorb more water back into our blood.

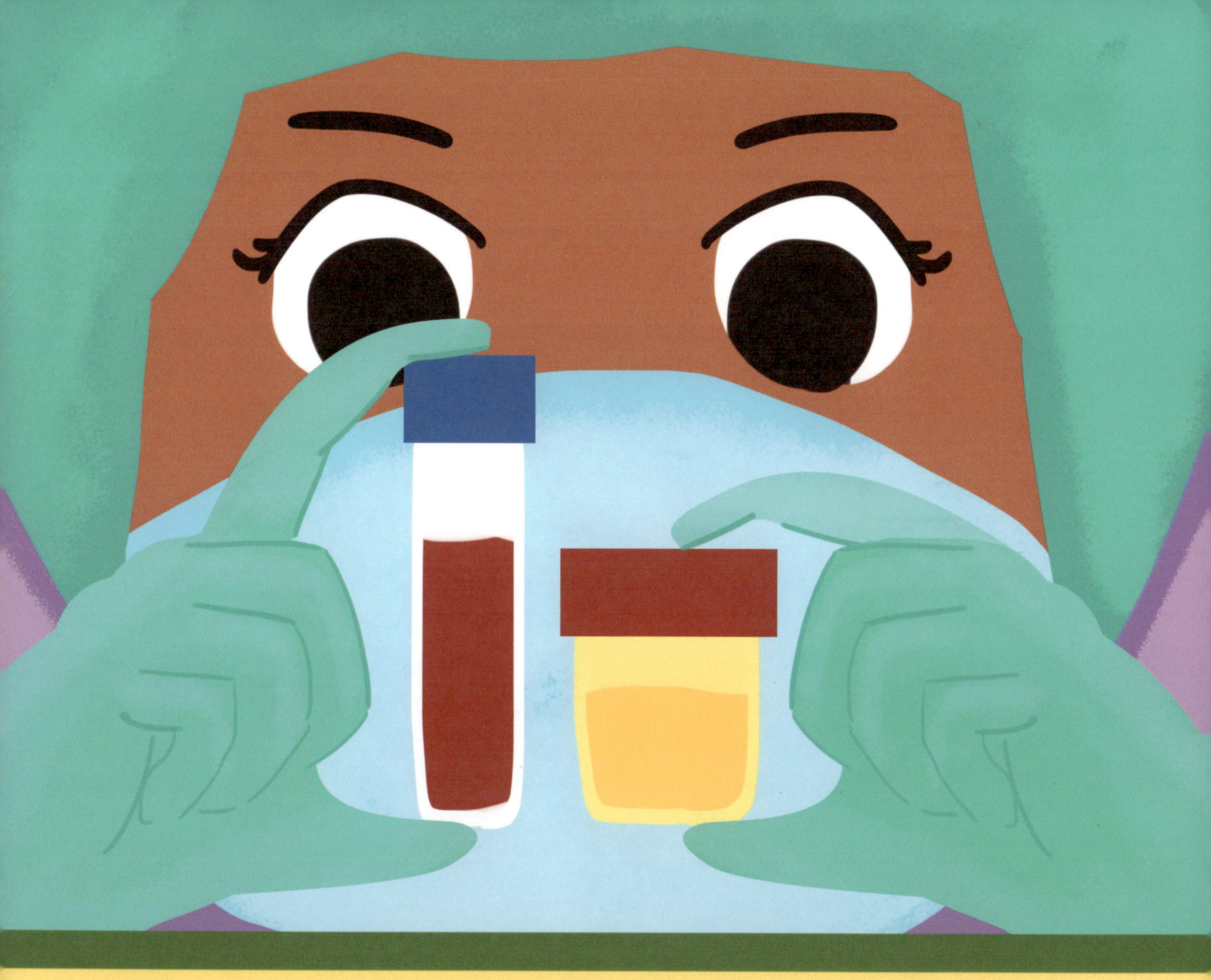

We can tell how well the kidneys are working by measuring the amount of **creatinine** in the *blood* and **protein** in the *urine.*

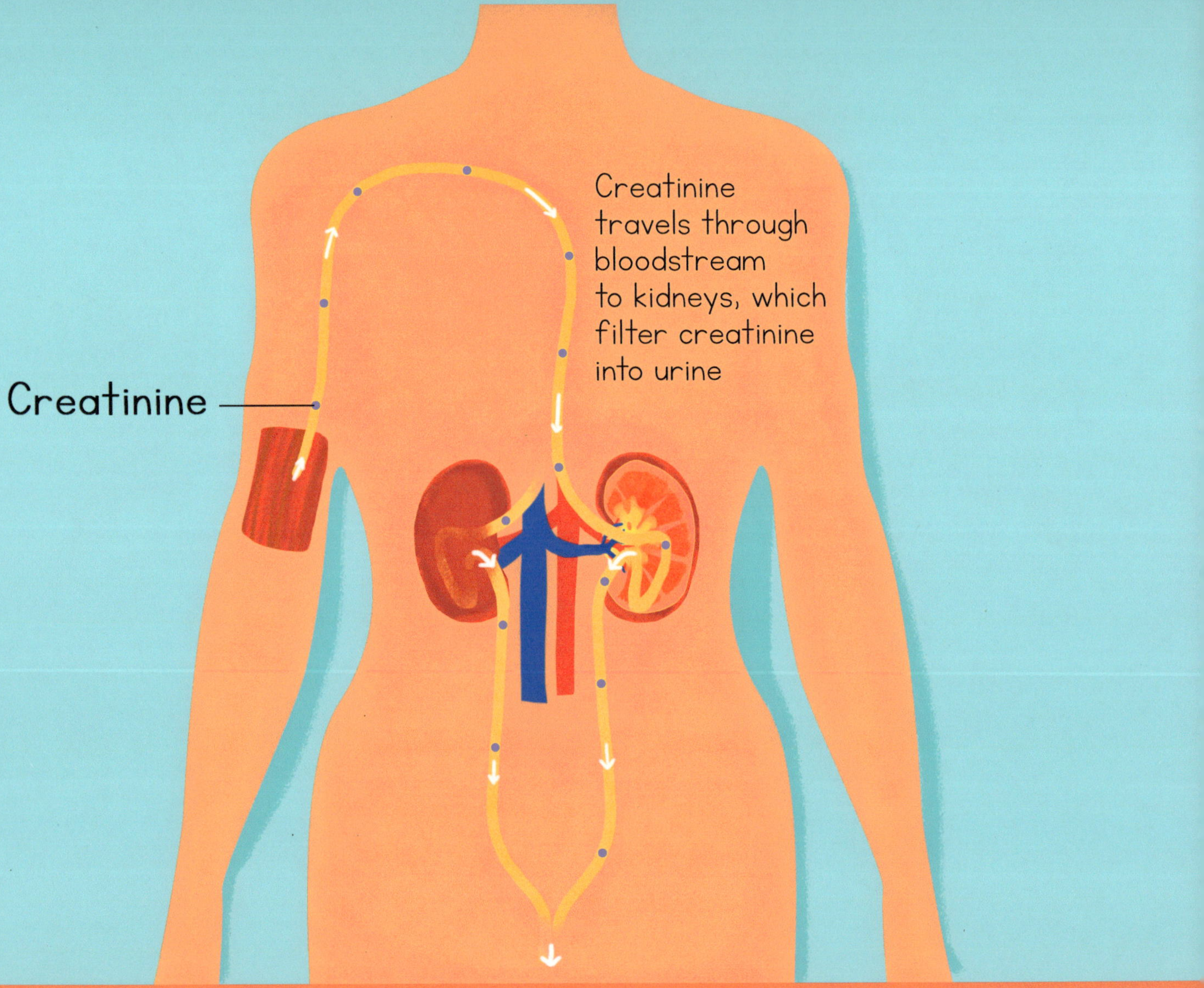

People with unhealthy kidneys can't remove a waste product called **creatinine** from their blood, so they will have high blood creatinine levels.

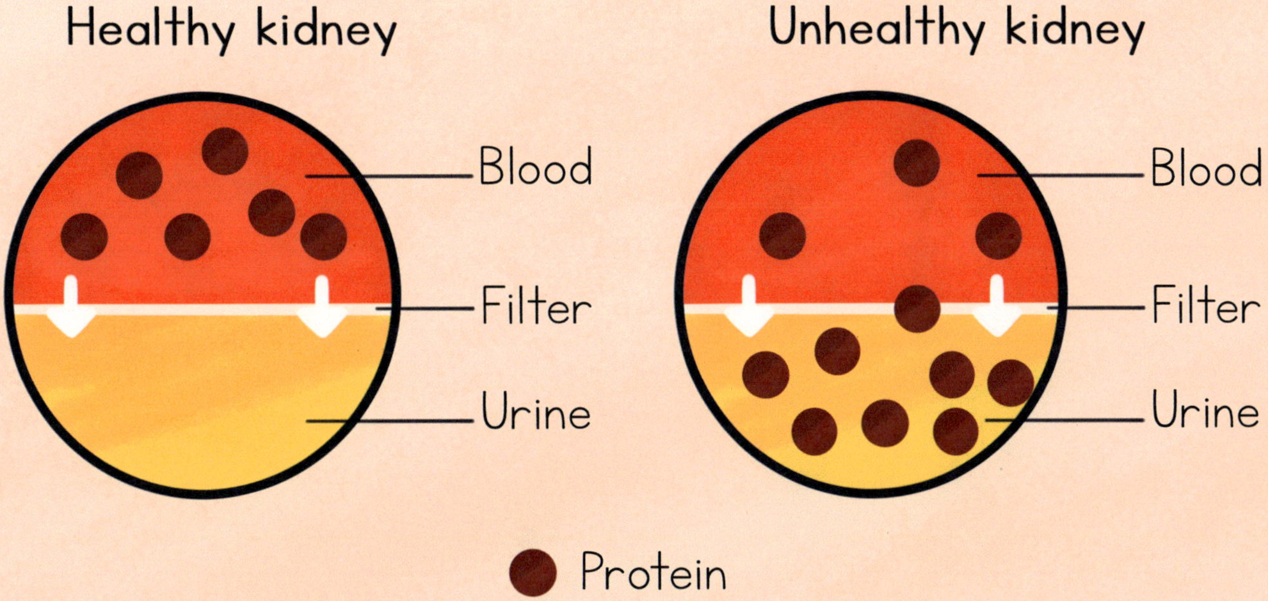

People with unhealthy kidneys can't prevent important **proteins** from leaving the blood into the urine, so they will have high urine protein levels.

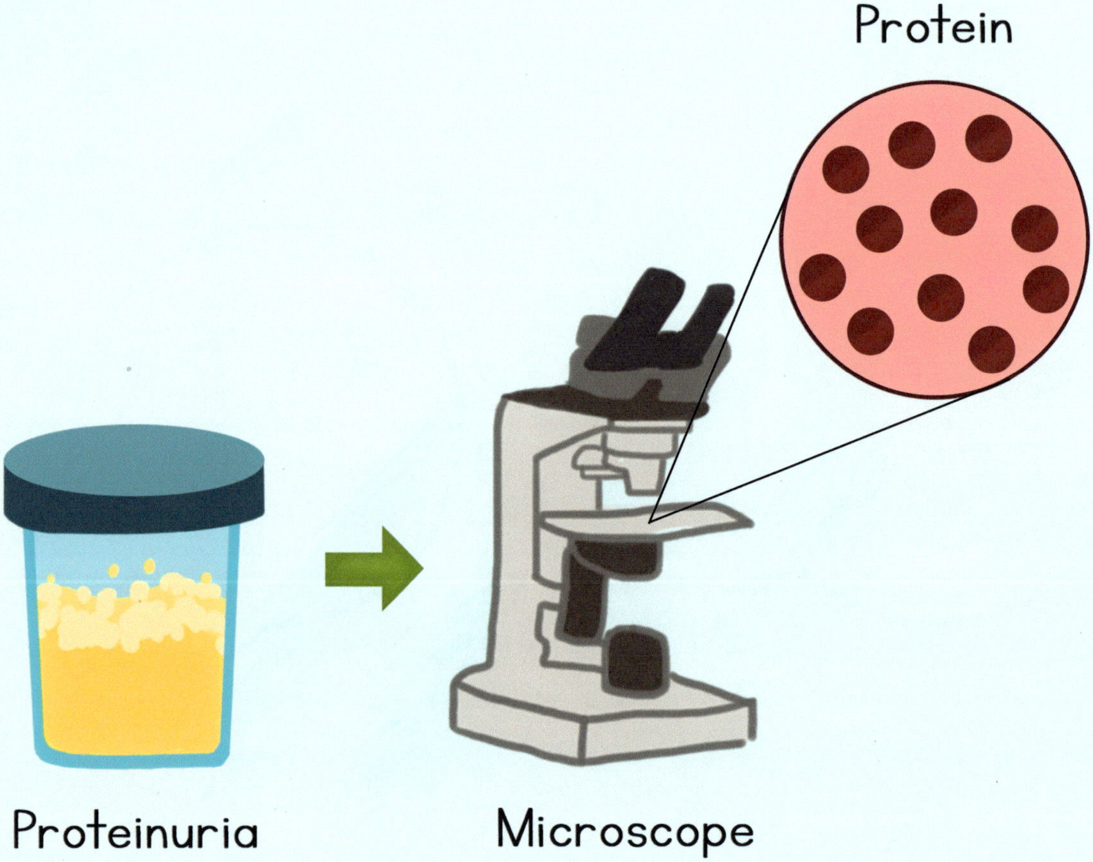

Protein in the urine, which is called **proteinuria**, causes urine to be foamy or bubbly.

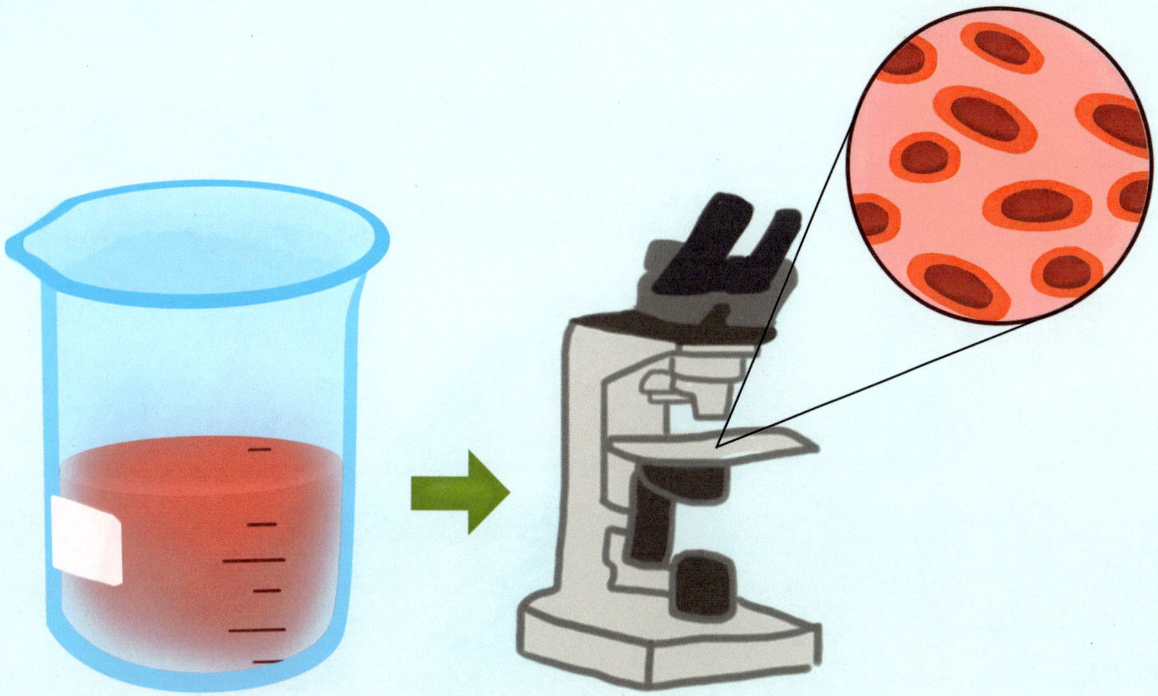

People with unhealthy kidneys may also have red blood cells in the urine. This is called **hematuria.**

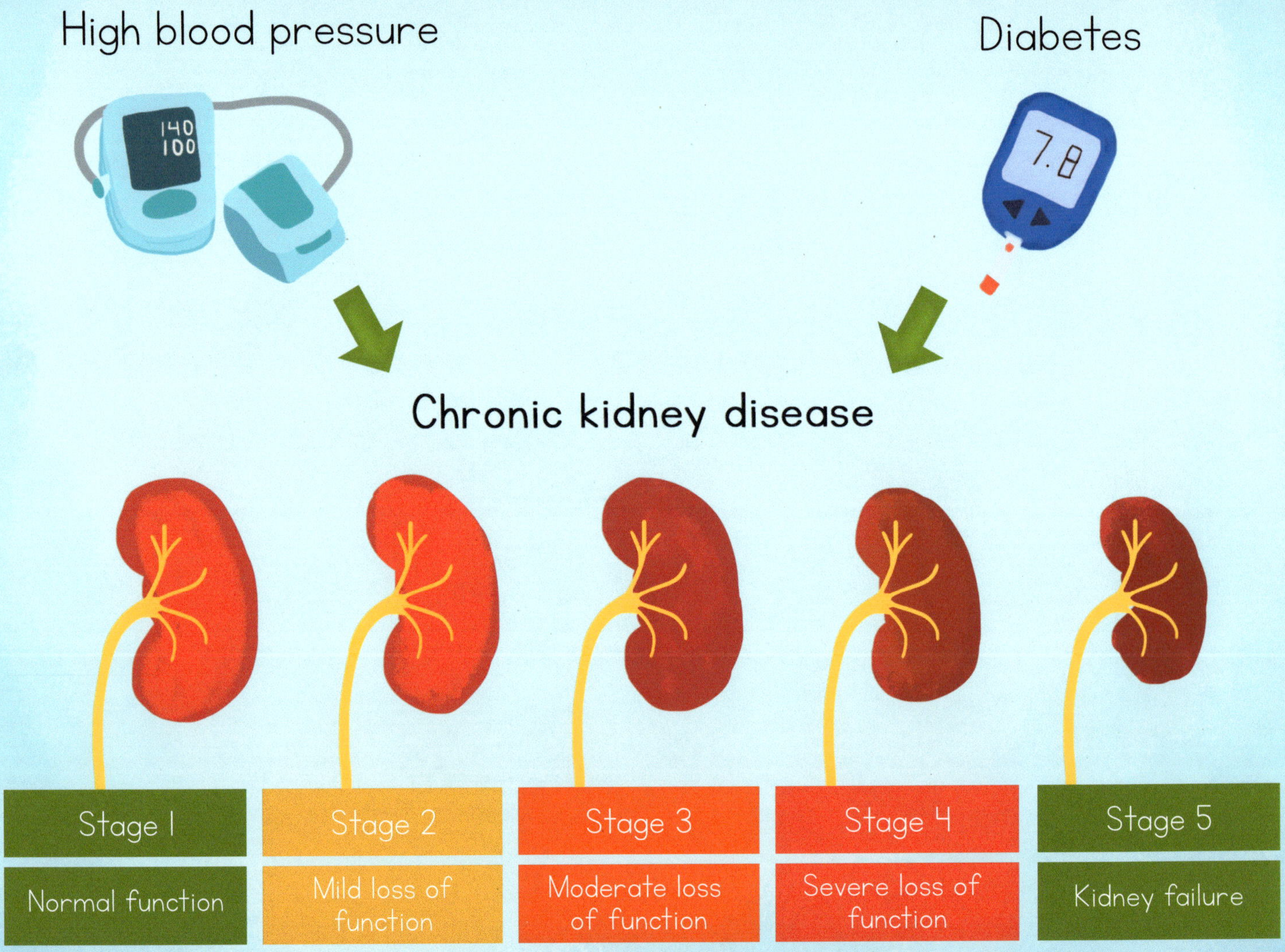

Some people develop kidney problems slowly over time. High blood pressure and diabetes can lead to **chronic kidney disease**.

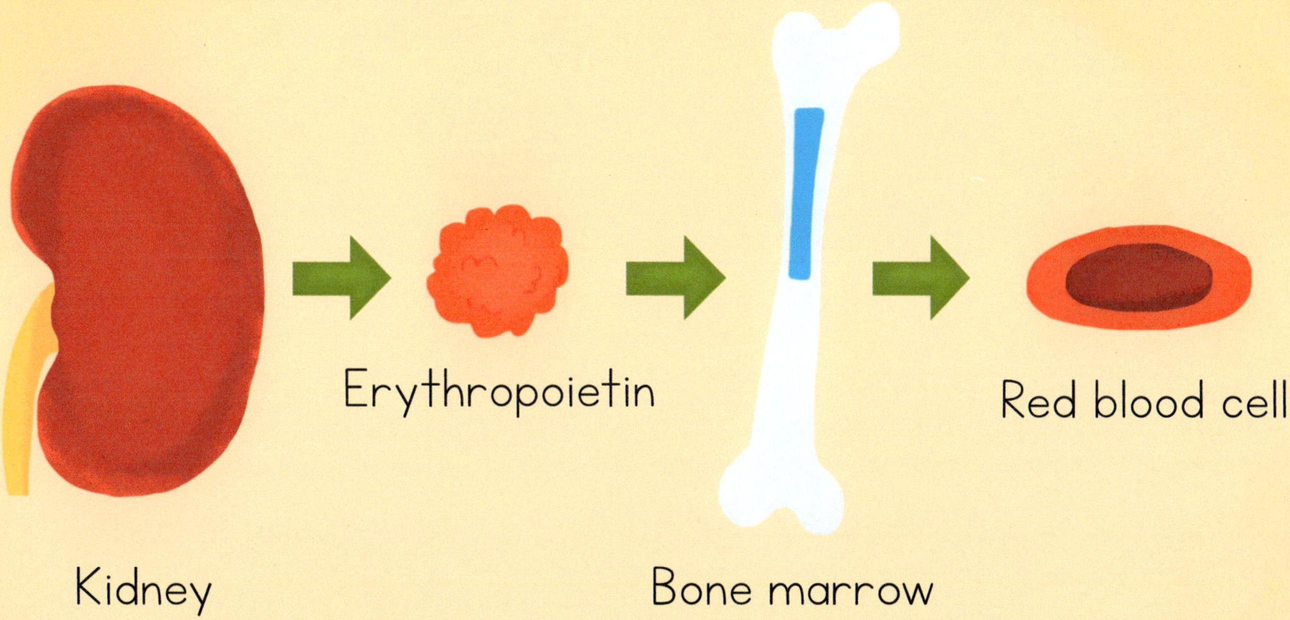

Chronic kidney disease can cause **anemia**, or low red blood cells, because the kidneys normally make a hormone (**erythropoietin**) that helps our body make red blood cells.

Causes of acute kidney injury

① Prerenal

Occurs when kidneys don't receive enough blood flow from the body

② Intrarenal

Occurs due to direct damage to the kidneys by inflammation, toxins, drugs, or infection

③ Postrenal

Occurs when the urinary tract below the kidneys is blocked

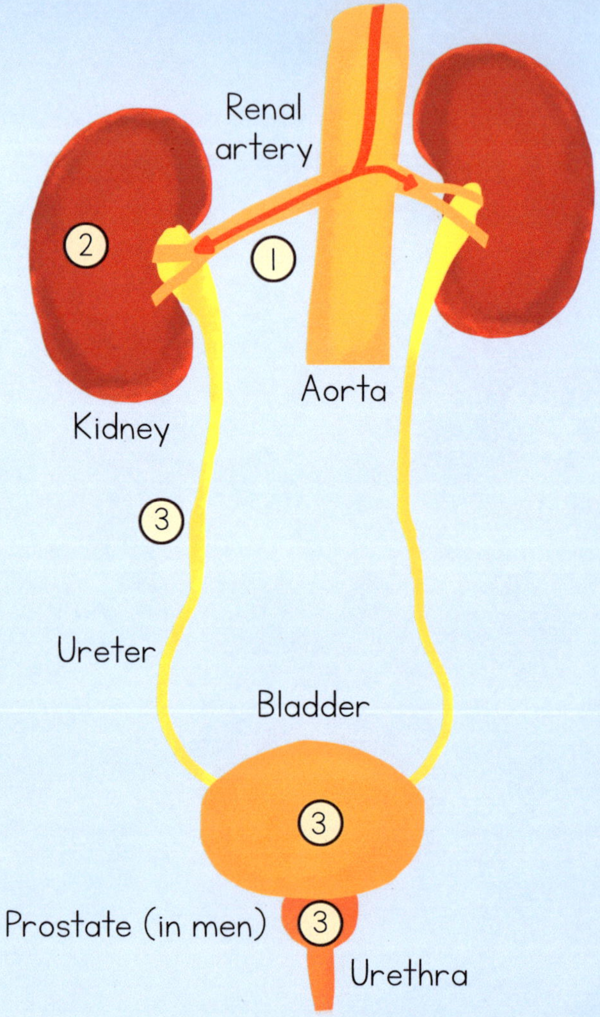

Other people can develop kidney problems suddenly, called **acute kidney injury**, which is divided into three categories: *prerenal*, *intrarenal*, and *postrenal*.

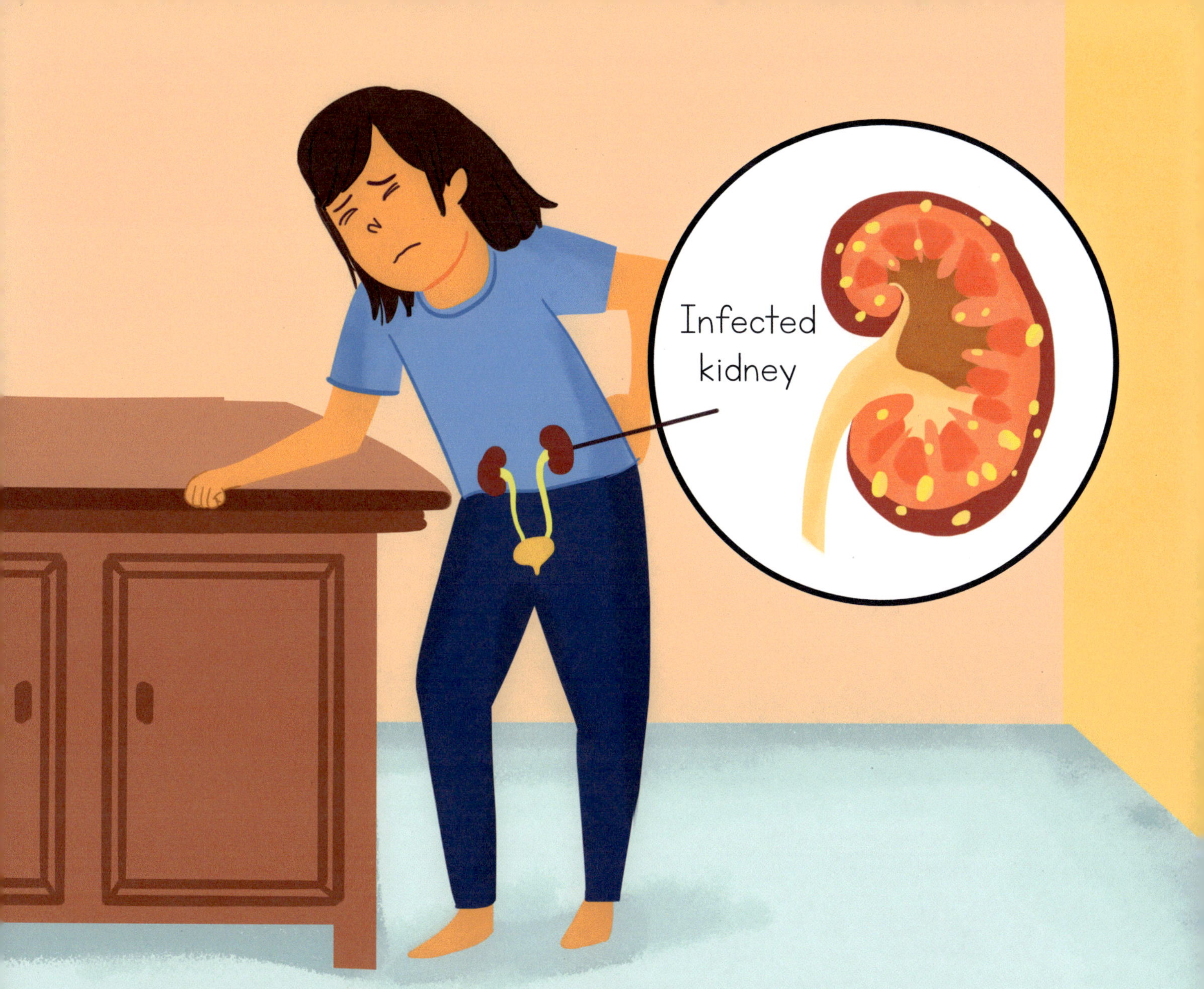

Like other organs in the body, the kidneys can sometimes become infected with bugs that make us sick. This is called **pyelonephritis**.

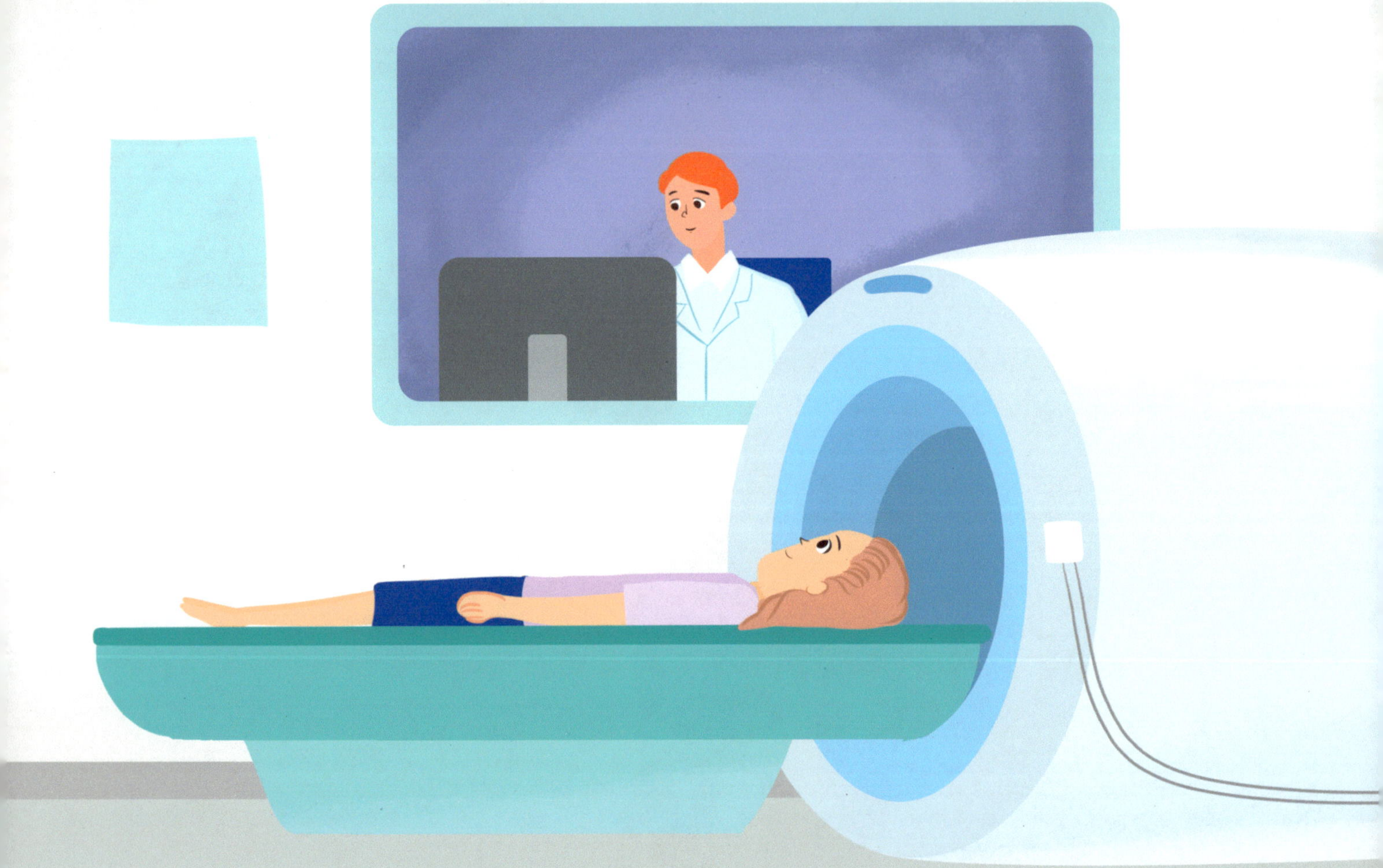

Doctors can diagnose certain kidney diseases using machines that can take pictures of the body, such as a **CT scanner** or **MRI scanner**.

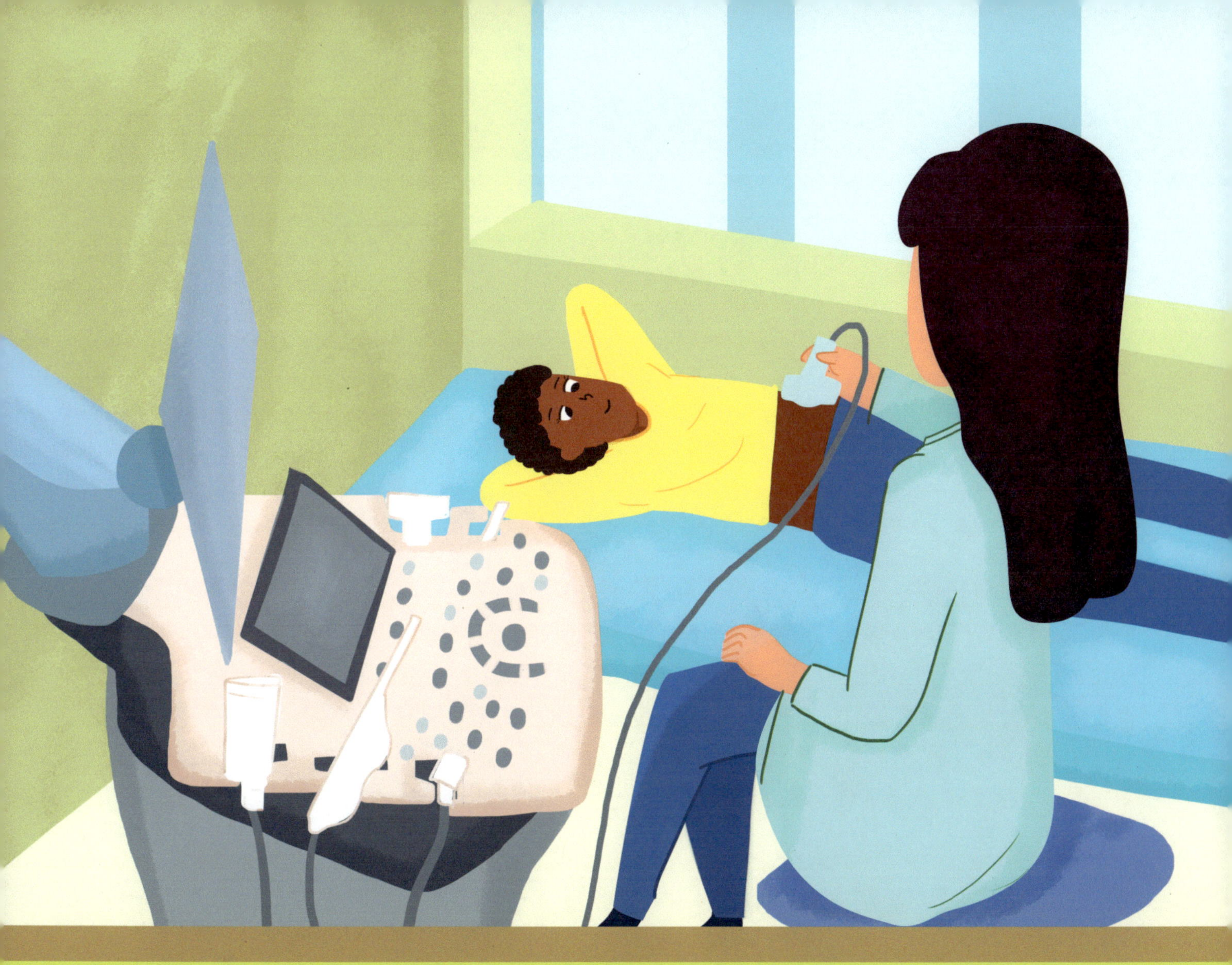

Doctors can also take pictures of the kidney using sound waves. This is called **kidney ultrasound**.

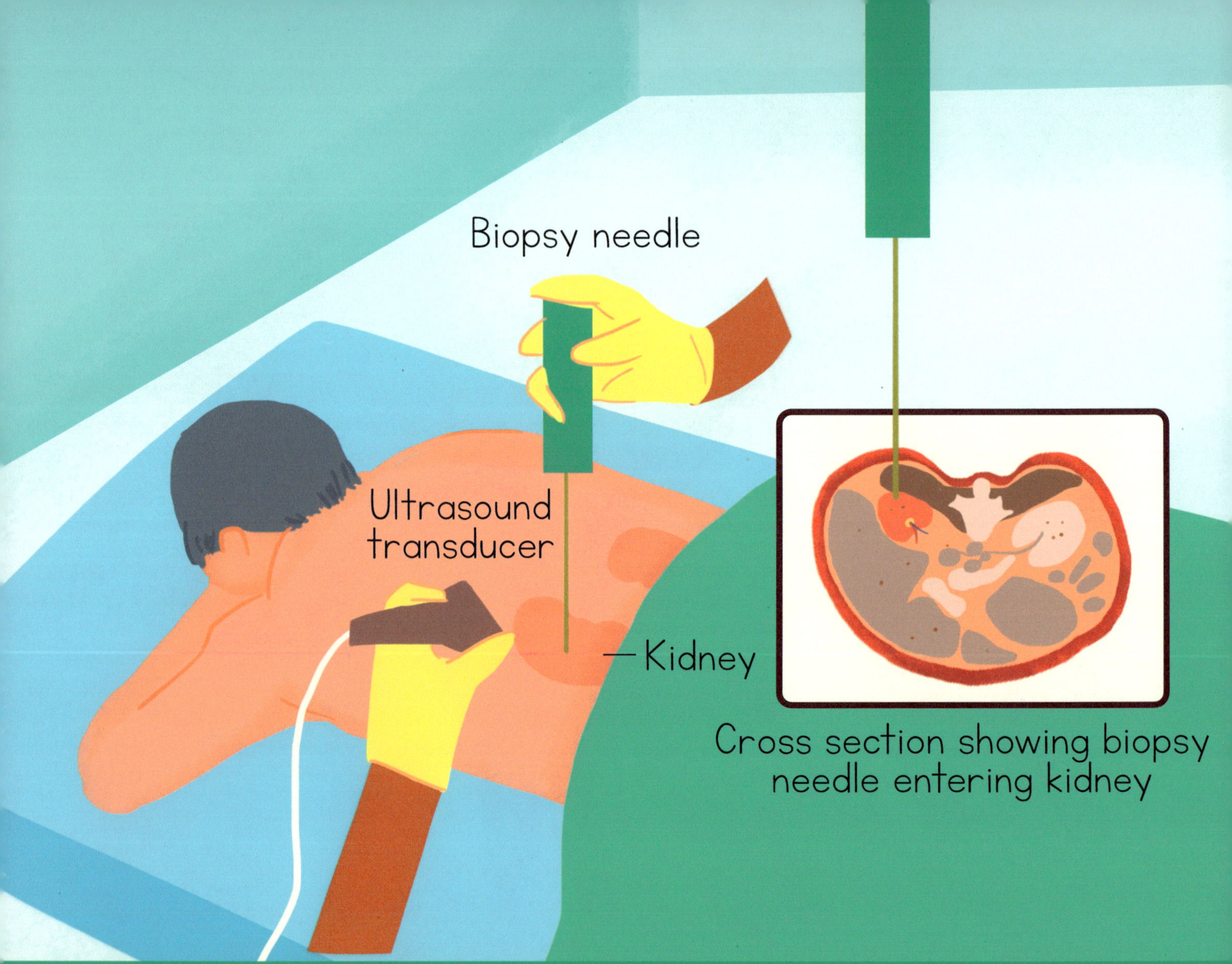

When the diagnosis is unclear, doctors can take a small sample of tissue, called a **biopsy**, from the kidney and look at it under a microscope.

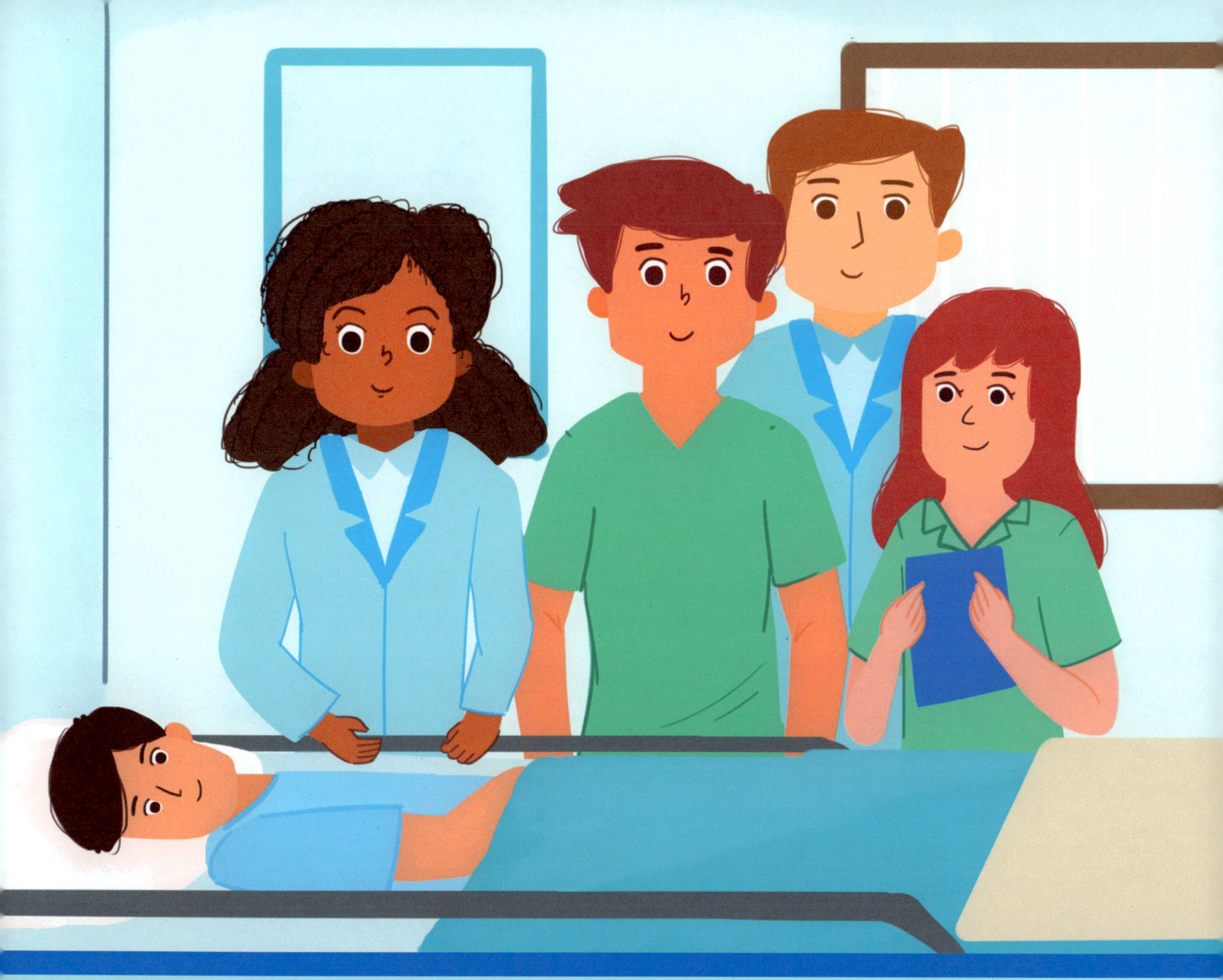

The good news is that nephrologists can treat kidney disease with different types of medications, procedures, and surgeries.

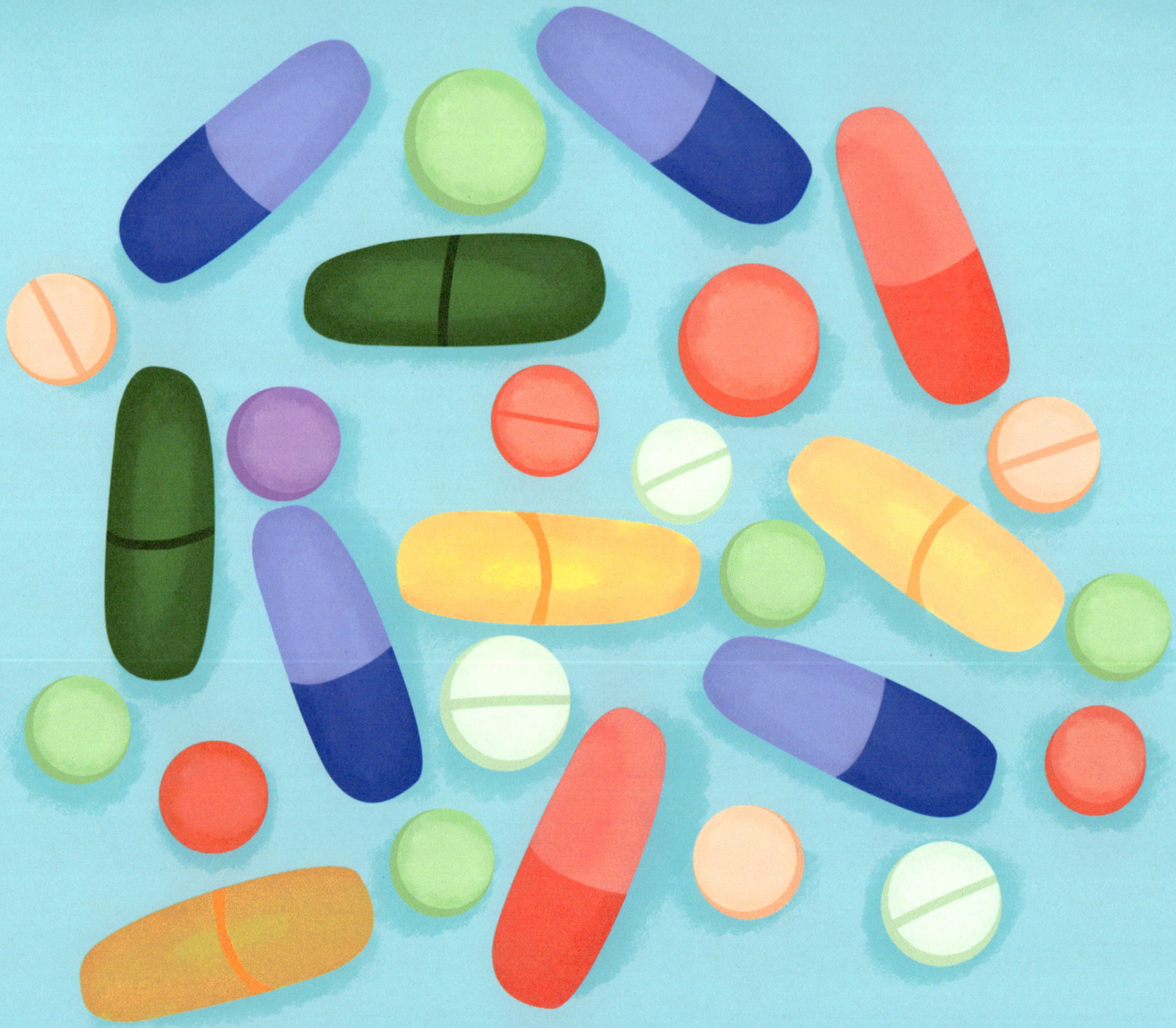

Patients with chronic kidney disease can take certain types of medications that lower blood pressure to slow the loss of kidney function.

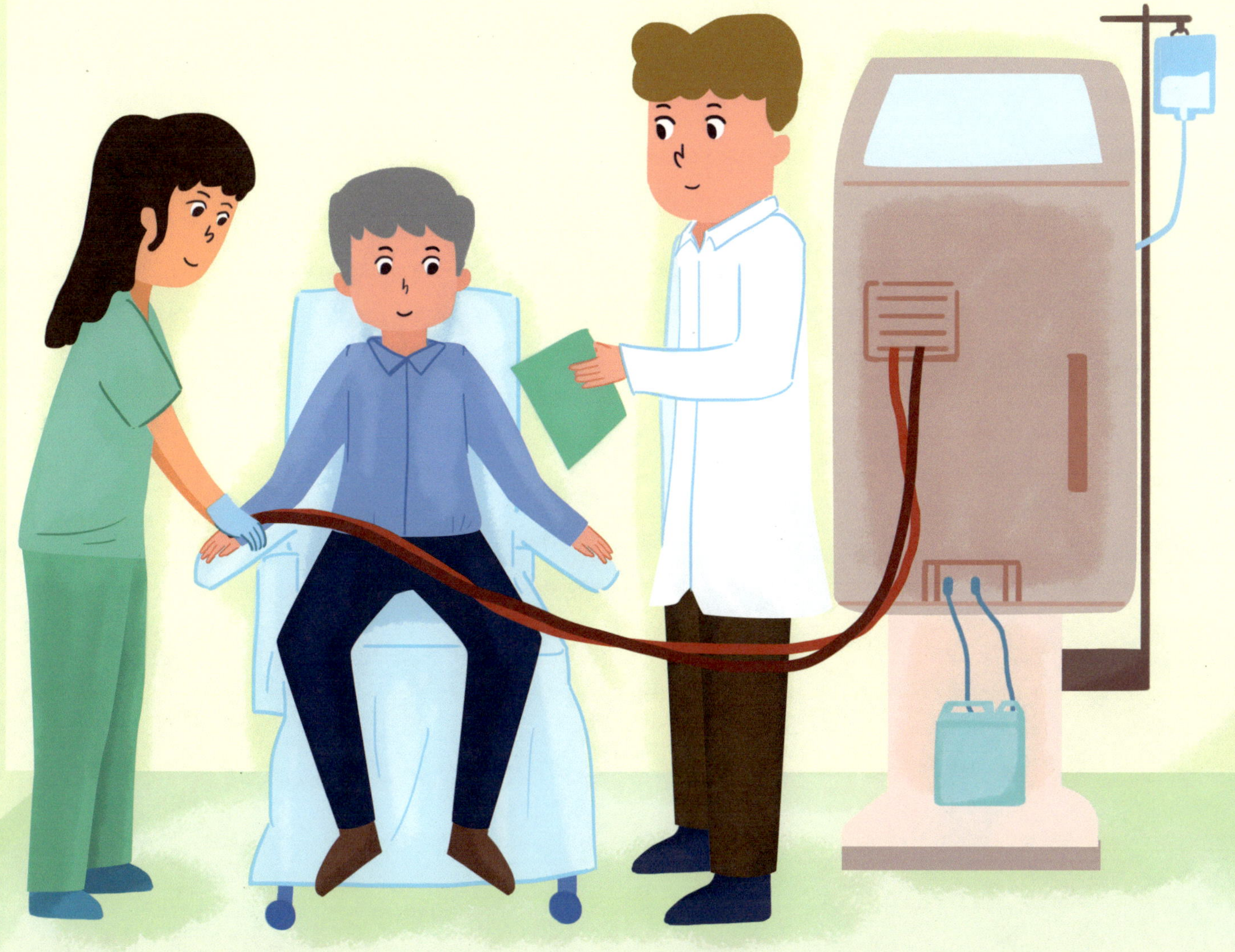

Patients with severe chronic kidney disease can be connected to a machine that filters their blood for them. This is called **dialysis**.

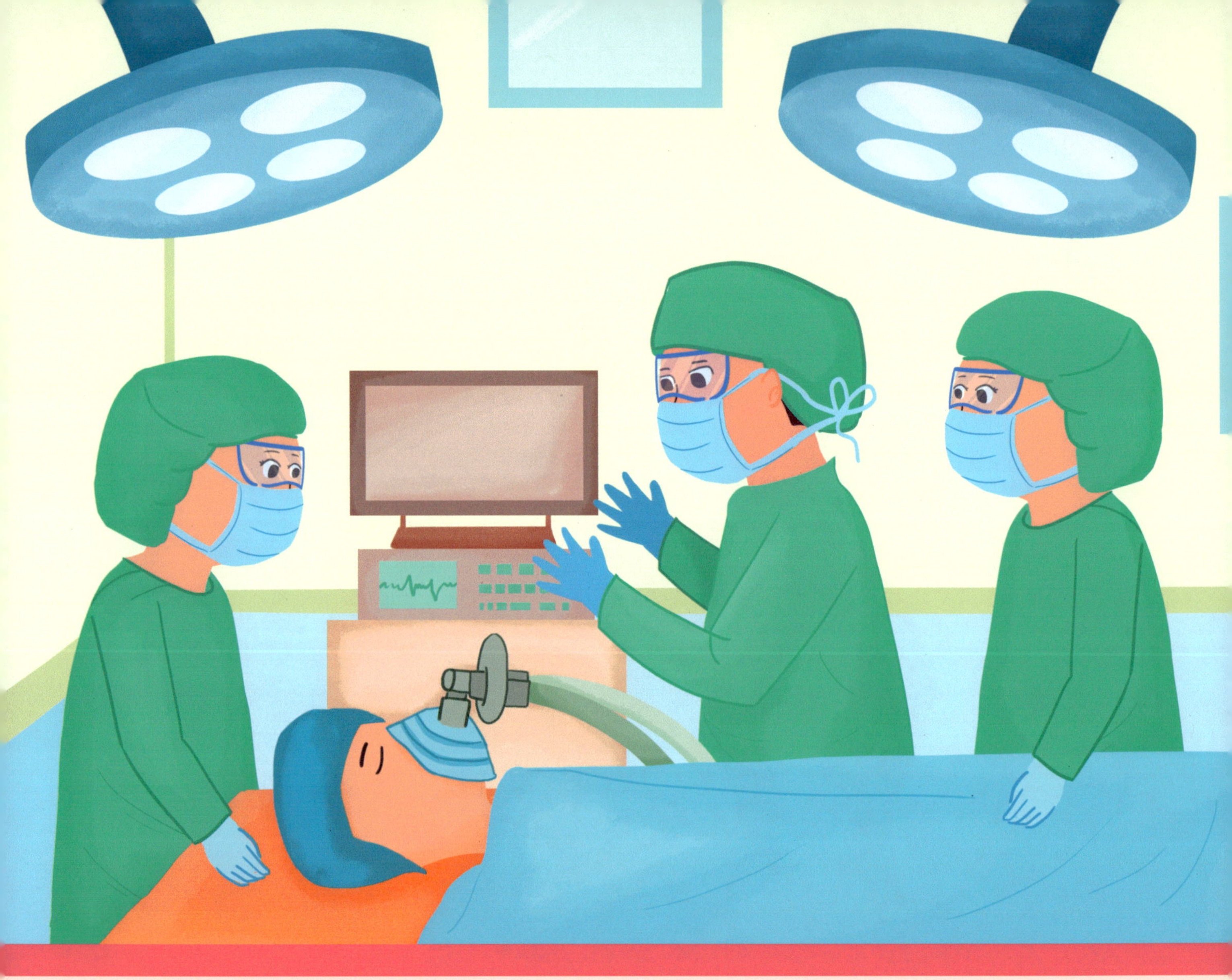

If needed, these patients can also receive a surgery called a **kidney transplant** that places a healthy kidney from a donor into their body.

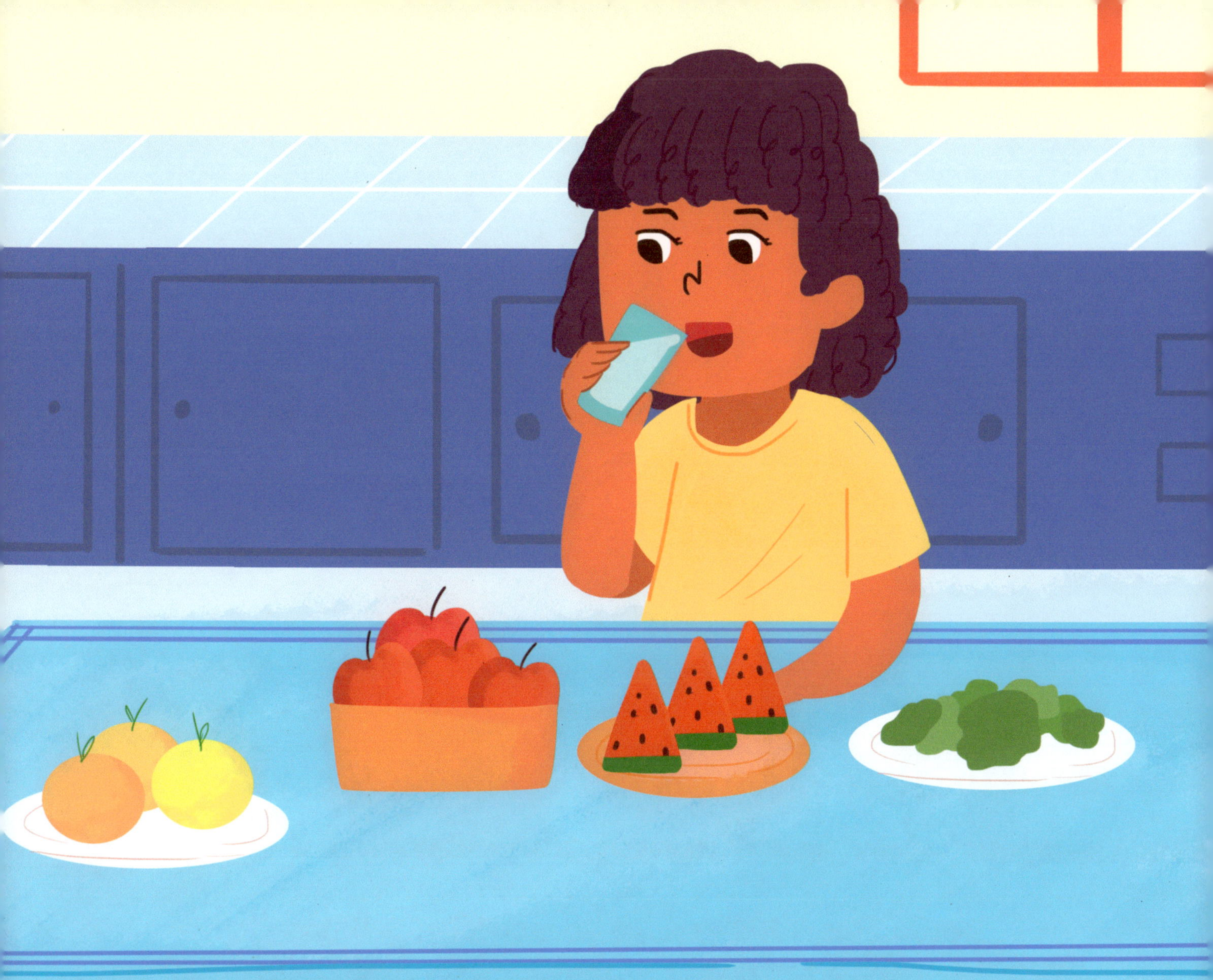

Drinking plenty of water, eating healthy foods, and exercising regularly helps keep our kidneys healthy.

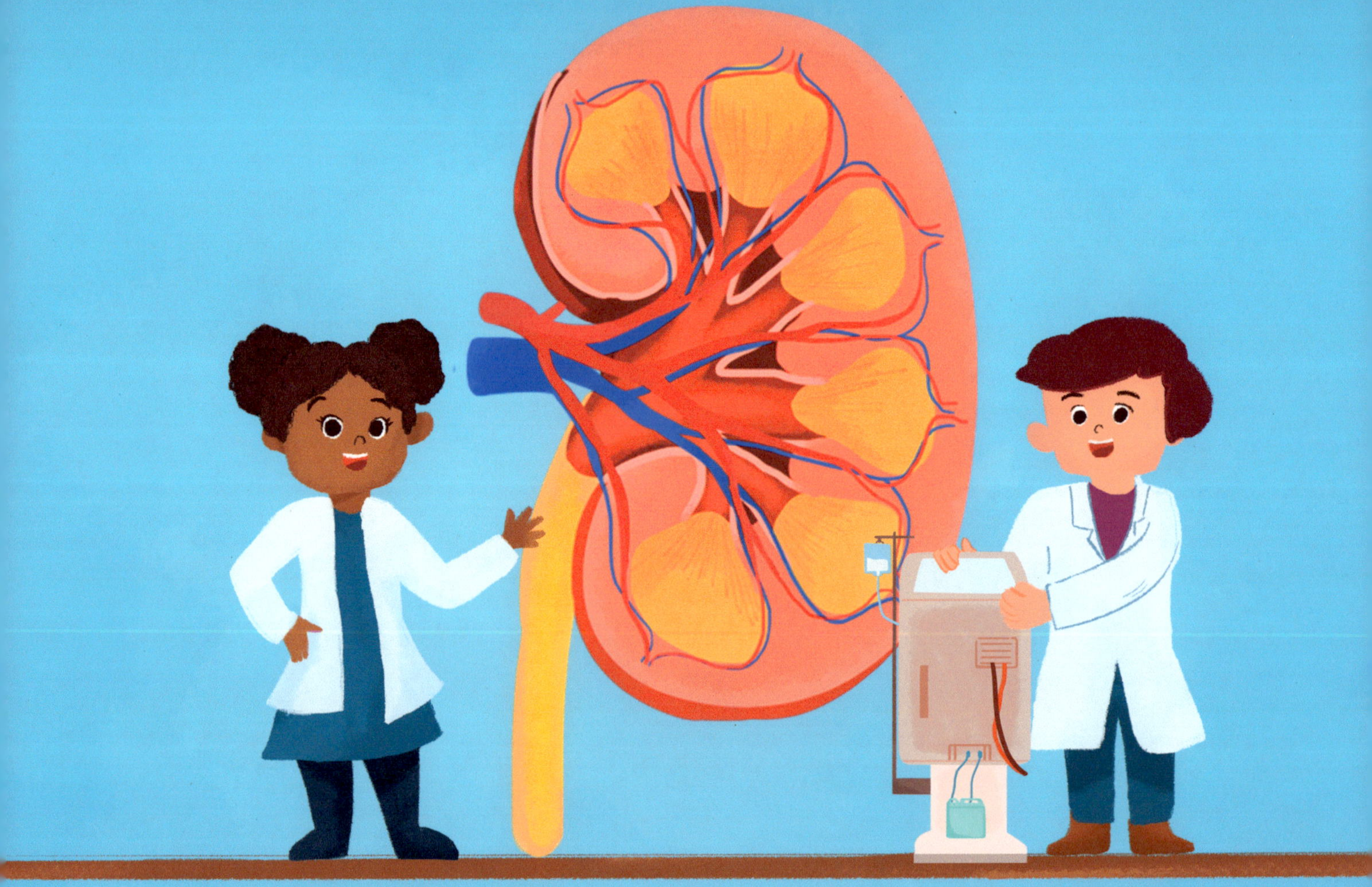

YOU'RE A FUTURE NEPHROLOGIST!

Glossary

Acute kidney injury: sudden decrease in kidney function due to prerenal, intrarenal, or postrenal cause

Anemia (uh-NEE-mee-uh): low levels of red blood cells in the body

Biopsy (BAI-aap-see): extraction of sample of tissue or cells from the body

Chronic kidney disease: slow decrease in kidney function over time; can be caused by medical conditions such as hypertension and diabetes

Creatinine (kree-A-tuh-neen): waste product made by our muscles

Dialysis (dai-A-luh-suhs): process of removing excess water and waste products from the blood in people whose kidneys no longer function normally

Erythropoietin (eh-ri-thruh-POY-tin): hormone made mainly by the kidneys that stimulates red blood cell production in the bone marrow

Glomerulus (gluh-MEHR-yuh-luhs): cluster of blood vessels located at the beginning of a nephron that filters blood

Hematuria (hee-muh-TUR-ee-uh): presence of blood in urine

Nephron (NEH-fraan): type of cell that makes up the kidneys

Proteinuria (prow-tee-NYUR-ee-uh): presence of protein in urine

Pyelonephritis (pai-uh-low-nuh-FRAI-tuhs): infection of the kidneys

Tubule (TOO-byool): the part of a nephron that collects blood

Kidney ultrasound (UHL-truh-sownd): test that creates pictures of the kidneys using sound waves

Vasopressin (va-suh-PREH-sn): hormone made by the brain that promotes retention of water by the kidneys

Answer Key

1. Below the ribcage; filter waste products from blood and make urine
2. Renal artery
3. Nephrons; glomerulus and tubule
4. Bowman's capsule, proximal tubule, loop of Henle, distal tubule, collecting duct
5. Renal vein
6. Light yellow
7. Vasopressin
8. Creatinine (in the blood) and protein (in the urine)
9. Proteinuria; hematuria
10. Hypertension and diabetes
11. Chronic kidney disease can cause anemia, or low red blood cells, because the kidneys normally make a hormone, called erythropoietin, that helps our body make red blood cells
12. Prerenal, intrarenal, and postrenal
13. Pyelonephritis
14. CT and MRI scan, kidney ultrasound, kidney biopsy
15. Dialysis

Medical School FOR KIDS™

About the Authors

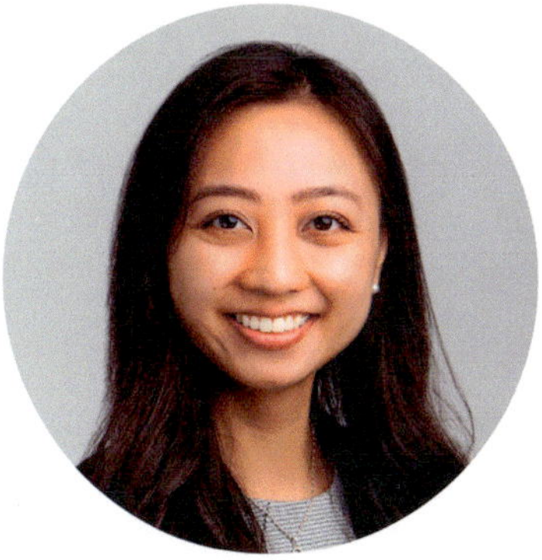

Betty Nguyen

Betty Nguyen was born in California but spent much of her childhood in Georgia, where she grew up on a chicken farm. She received a bachelor's degree in Biology from UCLA, where she received a full-ride Gates Millennium Scholarship through the Bill & Melinda Gates Foundation. Betty also received a full-tuition scholarship to attend medical school at the University of California, Riverside. Outside of work, Betty is a certified yoga instructor and licensed scuba diver. She also enjoys journalistic writing, cycling, and walking her two dogs in her free time.

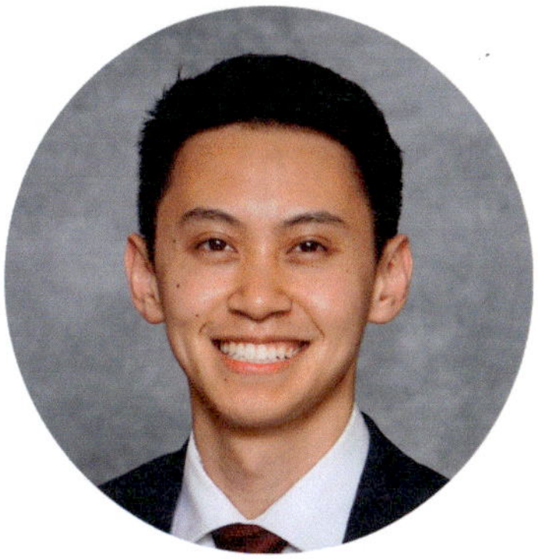

Brandon Pham

Brandon Pham was born and raised in California. He received a bachelor's degree in Microbiology, Immunology, and Molecular Genetics from UCLA, where he was a national Goldwater Scholar. He graduated from Stanford Medical School and is currently completing his residency in ophthalmology at the Bascom Palmer Eye Institute in Miami, Florida. Brandon spent many years teaching for several national test-preparation companies and is passionate about medical education for students of all ages. In his free time, Brandon enjoys traveling, playing tennis, and distance running.

Check out the rest of the books in our series!

Website: mdforkids.org

Instagram: @md.for.kids

Medical School FOR KIDS™